THE UN-DIET

*The Ultimate Mindset Journal
to Living Beyond Diets*

STACEY STEDMAN

outskirts
press

Outskirts Press, Inc.
http://www.outskirtspress.com

ISBN: 978-1-9772-3714-9

Outskirts Press and the "OP" logo are trademarks belonging to Outskirts Press, Inc.

PRINTED IN THE UNITED STATES OF AMERICA

Author's Note

All information in this book is for informational purposes only. This information is based on my personal health coaching opinion and in no way takes advise away from a professional Doctor or professional nutritionist. Please consult a doctor or nutritionist before beginning any nutrition program.

Day 1

Hello, hello! I'm so excited to have you here with me.

Welcome to day one of the Un-diet. There is so much more to losing weight than WHAT we are eating.

Yes, if you go through a fast-food drive-through every day, drink sodas, tons of alcohol, eat all the sugar that you can get your hands on, you will have a VERY hard time losing pounds.

But if you eat pretty healthy for the most part and keep not-so-healthy stuff as an "every once in a while," yet you struggle with losing weight and keeping it off, you've come to the right place.

I'm going to be sharing some information with you that may be the exact shift you've been looking for.

This is meant to be read every day, focusing on each day's task one day at a time. This gives our brain time to feel safe and secure to keep going.

When we are too overwhelmed with information, our limbic (emotional brain) takes over and possibly our survival brain, and we may go into fight-or-flight mode and not get what we want out of this.

I want you to have time to process and work on new information to help set yourself up for a positive mindset and habit change.

I will not be giving you a specific diet or meal plan.

I will not tell you to eliminate certain foods.

I will invite you to follow me on Facebook at The Un-Diet, where I'll share recipes and meal ideas.

I will be teaching you to get in tune with your body by fueling it properly, listening to your hunger cues, checking your emotions, and being in your neocortex brain (calm thinking brain) before you eat.

Every day you'll have a CTA (Call To Action), you must participate to get the results you're looking for. I promise you, if you sit on the sidelines and read your daily tasks but don't participate, you will stay exactly where you are.

Today's CTA:

This book is designed as a journal you can write in. Goals and tasks that are written down tend to stick a little better.

If you haven't written in a journal since you were a teenager, get comfortable and embrace this commitment to yourself.

Draw a line vertically down the journal page. Today you are going to write down on the left side of the paper the time and every item of food and drink that crosses your lips. On the right side you're going to write down a quick note on how you were FEELING when you ate or drank it.

Eat what you normally eat and pay attention to your feelings. Are you hungry, stressed, depressed, upset, tired, etc.

Embrace your journal and logging daily.

_____
_____
_____
_____
_____
_____
_____
_____
_____
_____
_____
_____
_____
_____

"Eat with love"

_____
_____
_____
_____
_____
_____
_____
_____
_____
_____
_____
_____
_____
_____
_____
_____
_____
_____
_____
_____
_____
_____
_____
_____
_____
_____
_____
_____

Day 2

Good morning! I hope you were able to track your food yesterday. We're going to play a little game of add-on for today.

You will be logging your foods and the feeling that goes along with it, but with today's CTA you will also be writing down any stomach or headache issues that you may have, before and after you eat. Scan your body every so often throughout the day to assess how you feel.

Being in control of your body is the most important thing you can do for your health, being mindful and aware of the foods that serve you and the foods that don't.

The fact that spinach is healthy doesn't mean it works for YOUR body.

For instance, some people can eat oatmeal in the mornings, feel completely satisfied and not hungry again until lunchtime and have tons of energy. Personally, if I eat oatmeal, I'm STARVING thirty minutes later, super hungry the entire day, and a little cranky.

I don't always track my nutrition anymore, but it's something I do when I'm feeling a bit out of control with my mindless snacking.

It's a great way to check yourself if you need to, but it's not required.

Now, this is only day two. Over the course of the month I will be getting into different things to try and why they may be good for your body and lifestyle.

Hang tight and keep logging, get in tune with that person inside of you that wants to be healthy and vibrant!

Please feel free to share your daily journal entries with me any time. You can send a picture of your daily journal to staceyhealthyfit@gmail.com or message me on Messenger.

"Nurture your soul"

_____
_____
_____
_____
_____
_____
_____
_____
_____
_____
_____
_____
_____
_____
_____
_____
_____
_____
_____
_____
_____
_____
_____
_____
_____

Day 3

There's a theory out there that it takes 21 days to build a new habit. It also takes 21 days to break a bad habit.

I'm not 100 percent sure about this, but I've done enough things in my life consistently for twenty-one days, and it really does help them stick.

That's why I want you to write everything you eat in this journal for the next thirty days. You will not be able to start shifting out of your current mindset about your nutrition without it.

Losing weight and keeping it off is 80 percent nutrition and 20 percent exercise.

We are going to continue writing everything down that we eat, how we feel, and if we notice any issues with anything.

Also, go ahead and note your daily exercise as well. I'd love to know what you're doing for movement, and it's important to your body and soul to move every day.

Your CTA for today:

Eat your food with presence, love, and appreciation, NO MATTER WHAT IT IS THAT YOU ARE EATING.

Seriously, be there with your meal, be present, notice your surroundings, use all your senses, don't be off in la-la land.

Feel love in your entire being when you eat.

Think thoughts of love and positivity, nothing else—no guilt, no shame, no stress. We will get to stress tomorrow.

Really enjoy your meals today.

_____

_____

_____

_____

_____

_____

_____

_____

_____

_____

_____

_____

_____

_____

_____

_____

_____

_____

_____

_____

_____

"My food is my fuel"

_____
_____
_____
_____
_____
_____
_____
_____
_____
_____
_____
_____
_____
_____
_____
_____
_____
_____
_____
_____
_____
_____
_____
_____
_____
_____
_____

Day 4

There is a connection between stress and metabolism. This is BIG.

The autonomic nervous system is responsible for digestive activity. There are two branches: the parasympathetic and the sympathetic.

The parasympathetic is known as the rest-and-digest response.

Our metabolic power goes up when this is activated, and this is the optimal state for digestion.

The sympathetic is known as fight or flight. This is our stress response. When we are stressed, our digestion shuts down. The classic textbook example is if a bear is chasing you after lunch, you won't be concerned about digesting your sandwich. The sympathetic nervous system acts efficiently in this stressed state to shut down digestion and direct blood flow out to your arms and legs for quick moving and your brain for quick thinking. The blood flow moves away from being able to digest your food in a stressed state.

This is a wonderful system in place for our survival. While most of us do not have to confront bears on our lunch hour, we do encounter stress.

On a physiological level your body doesn't differentiate between the bear chasing you or your boss yelling at you or getting stuck in a traffic jam. One is life threatening, and the others are not, but guess what? On a physiological level they are the same, they all trigger the body to shut off digestion and store fat, which decreases our metabolic power.

The hormone cortisol is released when we are stressed out, and increased cortisol in your system leads to fat accumulation, mainly around the midsection. Do you gain more weight around your belly?

People who tend to gain weight around the belly likely experience chronic low-level stress, so if you are or know someone that has smaller legs or smaller arms and tend to gain weight in the belly, that's most likely the result of stress.

If your body is in even a low-level stress state most of the time, you may lose a few pounds here and there but ultimately no amount of calorie counting or running will get you where you want to go.

Your CTA for today:

Recognize when you are stressed. What do you do about it? Write it in your journal.

_____

_____

_____

_____

_____

_____

_____

_____

_____

_____

_____

_____

_____

_____

_____

_____

_____

_____

_____

_____

_____

_____

_____

_____

_____

_____

_____

"Stressed is desserts spelled backwards"

_____

_____

_____

_____

_____

_____

_____

_____

_____

_____

_____

_____

_____

_____

_____

_____

_____

_____

_____

_____

_____

_____

_____

_____

_____

_____

_____

_____

_____

_____

Day 5

Secret to burning more fat:

RELAX.

Why is relaxing important? Digestive stress is about 25 percent WHAT you eat, and 75 percent WHO we are being.

Who are you being when you eat or when you are healing?

Are you moving at warp speed?

Constantly eating on the go?

Multitasking during the meal?

Engaging in gossip?

These are all ways in which we feed the stress response.

Eating under stress is not only commonplace, it's also socially acceptable and often a prerequisite for managing a job, dealing with family, or having a life.

When do we feel stressed? Mostly when we are moving too fast.

Stress is the opposite of relaxation.

If you've worked for a stronger metabolism (or you've been trying to heal your body) but have not achieved success, there's one basic reason.

YOU ARE MOVING TOO FAST!

When moving through life too fast we inevitably eat fast, which destroys our metabolism and creates digestive upset. It results in meals eaten under a physiologic stress response, which diminishes our calorie-burning power.

The slower you eat, the faster you metabolize. The more relaxed you are throughout your day, the more energy you will have.

That late-afternoon slump that happens is because we are sprinting throughout the day, and then we have to rest and recuperate. We get sleepy, foggy brain. We can't do anymore, and that's when we end up bingeing or turning to something that will provide us with pleasure, because we're not getting enough pleasure throughout the day. We're just stressing.

Let this part sink in:

You can eat the healthiest meal on the planet, but if you eat it in a stressed out, anxious state, your digestion is dramatically diminished.

Here is the scientific perspective of what happens when we are stressing: salivary enzyme content in the mouth is reduced; the breakdown of protein, fat, and carbs in the stomach is impaired. Blood flow to the small intestines is decreased as much as fourfold, which translates into not being able to assimilate vitamins, minerals, and other nutrients, as well.

Have you ever had the experience of eating a full meal and still being hungry, like you just can't get satisfied? When has that happened to you?

Here is your solution to calming your stress BEFORE you eat anything:

The 5-5-7 breath.

Before you eat, ask yourself, "Am I about to eat under stress?" If the answer is yes, pause, and take ten long, slow, deep breaths:

Inhale for the count of 5 filling lungs to two-thirds capacity.

Hold for 5.

Exhale to the count of 7.

Your eyes can be open or closed. You must sit comfortably, spine straight, and feet flat on the floor. As you continue doing this conscious breathing, use a steady rhythm and scan the senses.

This is two minutes of relaxation that can be done anywhere, anytime.

Breathing before and during your meals is a great way to become a relaxed eater and boost your metabolic power.

You can also do this breathing exercise in your car, at work, and before bed (my personal favorite). Even when there is chaos going on around you, pay attention to who you are being. Can you relax into the chaos?

Some people say, "But if I'm relaxed, I won't get as much done." Relaxing isn't necessarily about non-doing, it's about who you are being.

Practice using conscious breath throughout the day and working in the rhythm of relaxation. You'll find that you are more focused, more productive, and more energized. It's very exhausting to be in a stressed state all the time. You use a lot of energy and still store a lot of fat.

Metabolism is really about heating the body, which is what burning calories means. When we eat the right foods we feed the furnace. The breath helps with the burn because it warms the body. Breathe in more oxygen, and you burn food more fully.

Did you know that we lose most of our weight through our breath? Eighty-four percent of fat loss is exhaled as carbon dioxide.

Simply by relaxing the breath—conscious breathing—your capacity for burning calories or burning fat goes up.

Your CTA:

Take notice and write down when you are stressed out. Incorporate the 5-5-7 breathing technique throughout the day, and continue writing in your journal.

_____

_____

_____

_____

_____

_____

_____

_____

_____

_____

_____

_____

_____

_____

_____

_____

_____

_____

_____

_____

_____

_____

_____

_____

_____

_____

"You've got this"

Day 6

I hope this past five days have been eye opening for you in regard to paying attention to your eating habits, your stress, your breathing, etc.

We are going to continue with all of that, as well as figuring out foods that give you energy. When you think of high-energy foods, what are your first thoughts?

At what time of day do you notice an energy crash?

I am going to give you a few different ways of eating to see how YOUR body responds best:

- ☛ Eating five to six small meals a day (between 200 and 300 calories) and not going longer than two to three hours between eating.
- ☛ Intermittent fasting (eating meals in a six- to eight-hour time frame)
- ☛ Eating three fairly large meals (500 to 600 calories each) with no snacking or anything else.

Here is a quick glance of the different ways of eating and why:

The theory behind eating five to six small meals a day with no more than two to three hours in between: your metabolism is in a constant state of "fire," and you don't fall into the blood-sugar roller-coaster. (Calories per meal are roughly between 200 and 300)

The theory behind eating three large, well-balanced meals and no snacking: your body has time to process and digest. You have a lot of food on your plate, which makes you feel happy and satisfied. Thinking about food and meal prep can be greatly diminished. (Calories per meal are roughly between 500 and 600)

The theory behind intermittent fasting (eating in a six- to eight-hour window), along with high protein and fat and very low carbs is that your body gets forced into being in a fat-burning stage, not a normal sugar-burning stage. It revs up the metabolism and uses the back stock of fat, because there's nothing else left. (You will quite possibly be eating only two meals a day, so be sure to get your daily calories in, you will have to add some healthy fats). This food plan is a tough one to stick to for the long term, but if you're interested, please do a little research before diving in. Please consult your Doctor before trying any new dietary program.

Your CTA for today:

After reading these food plans, which one resonates with you most?

Was there one in particular that excited you?

Did you want to test out all of them over the next three weeks or pick one and stick to it?

Which one would you like to try first?

You will want to do each one for at least four to six days, really getting in tune with how your body is feeling.

You will continue logging your food (and drinks) and the feelings you have with both.

_____

_____

_____

_____

_____

_____

_____

_____

_____

_____

_____

_____

_____

_____

_____

_____

_____

_____

"I am in tune with my body"

_____
_____
_____
_____
_____
_____
_____
_____
_____
_____
_____
_____
_____
_____
_____
_____
_____
_____
_____
_____
_____
_____
_____
_____
_____
_____
_____

Day 7

Focus on our health from the inside out, not the outside in.

What does that mean?

When we focus on our health from the inside out, we are doing the internal work first. We are slowing down, becoming more aware and present of the body we've been given. We need to be able to look in the mirror and love that person we see looking back at us.

When we focus on our health from the outside in, we've started a diet and or exercise program, we're doing the work for an end result of how we want to look, whether it be weight loss, getting more toned, building muscle, etc. We might be eating a diet that we hate or is too strict, which in turn means we may be a bit miserable and/or resentful.

We may be liking what we are seeing from the outside, but how are we feeling on the inside?

How is your internal dialogue when you look in the mirror?

What you are saying to yourself matters.

Is it positive or negative?

Today your CTA is to notice what things go through your head when you look in the mirror. Just notice, are they positive or are they negative? How many times a day do you think something bad about yourself?

The best way to reverse a negative thought is to say/think of three positive things about yourself EVERY time that negative thought crossed your mind. (You may be busy today reversing those negative thoughts, and that's OK).

_____

_____

_____

_____

_____

_____

_____

_____

_____

_____

_____

_____

_____

_____

_____

_____

_____

_____

_____

_____

_____

_____

_____

"A positive mind is a positive body"

_____
_____
_____
_____
_____
_____
_____
_____
_____
_____
_____
_____
_____
_____
_____
_____
_____
_____
_____
_____
_____
_____
_____
_____
_____

Day 8

Our goals can seem distant, and change can be overwhelming, but when you choose to focus your efforts on taking one step toward a healthier, happier you every day, even the biggest challenges seem easier to get through.

What I really want you to focus on is how you feel. What feels in line with you?

If it's something you are dreading, don't do it, if it's something you are curious and excited about, then by all means, give it a go.

Before bed in the evening or when you wake up in the morning, set one health intention for the next day.

1. Prepare: Make your lunch for work the night before.
2. Nourish: Wake up fifteen minutes earlier to make time to enjoy a nourishing breakfast at home before a busy day.
4. Limber up: Take five to ten minutes in the morning to stretch, meditate, or go through a short yoga sequence.
5. Keep calm: Leave for work five minutes earlier to get there stress-free, with time to spare.
6. Dress up: Put on an outfit that makes you feel confident. Throw on those pearls, playful scarf, or earrings.
8. Hydrate: Drink a glass of water before each meal throughout the day.
9. Breathe: Go for a twenty-minute walk on your lunch break to get your steps in and breathe in some fresh air.
10. Go green: Grab a fruit or vegetable for an afternoon pick-me-up.
11. Connect: Call a family member or friend to catch up or simply talk about your day.
12. Be mindful: Eat your dinner at a table without distractions. Every family member's phone should be away from the dinner table, upside down, and silent.

Your CTA today:

How many of these things do you already do, and how many of them will you start incorporating daily?

_____

_____

_____

_____

_____

_____

_____

_____

_____

_____

_____

_____

_____

_____

_____

_____

_____

_____

_____

_____

_____

_____

_____

_____

_____

"I am always learning"

Day 9

YOU CANNOT GET A POSITIVE OUTCOME WITH A NEGATIVE MIND.

Today we are decluttering our minds. It is one of the most important things to declutter.

Our minds can be filled with so much negative talk, self-deprecating thoughts, and thinking too much about things that happened in the past or may happen in the future.

Your CTA today and from here on out is to bring yourself back to the present moment when your thoughts go astray. Don't beat yourself up, just kindly bring yourself back to the present time.

Also, every time a negative thought runs through your head, stop yourself by saying "I know what I don't want; what is it that I do want?" and then think of three positive things to change that negative thought pattern.

_____

_____

_____

_____

_____

_____

_____

_____

_____

_____

_____

_____

_____

_____

_____

_____

_____

_____

_____

_____

"Being present is a present"

_____

_____

_____

_____

_____

_____

_____

_____

_____

_____

_____

_____

_____

_____

_____

_____

_____

_____

_____

_____

_____

_____

_____

_____

_____

_____

_____

_____

_____

Day 10

Hunger, Appetite and Emotional Eating

To do list today:

Record your observations by writing in your journal.

Each time you feel compelled to eat, take note and answer the following questions:

- Where do I feel hungry?
- Do I feel hungry in my stomach?
- Is this a desire to eat?
- Is this desire to eat triggered by habit, emotion, feelings, time of day, circumstances, or the setting?
- Do I truly feel physical hunger?

Hunger vs. Appetite

True hunger is a physical feeling that results from a combination of hormones, your metabolic process, and the amount of available fuel. It is characterized by a feeling, often in the stomach, and sometimes in the lower part of your chest.

It can be accompanied by weakness, a gnawing pain, churning in the stomach, a headache, lightheadedness, or even stomach contractions that create a desire to eat.

True hunger is different from appetite. Hunger is a physical drive to eat, while appetite is often psychological. Here's the kicker: just about any type of fuel alleviates real hunger. If you were stranded on a deserted island and you were truly hungry, you could take care of that feeling by eating a pile of bugs, but you might still crave a certain type of food—that's your appetite.

Hunger is fixed by fuel, whether it's healthy or not. If you're truly hungry, then broccoli, carrots, or some other healthy food would take care of it.

What is going on when we eat but are not truly hungry?

When we feel an overwhelming desire to eat but in our minds, we think, "Gosh, I shouldn't be hungry," that is appetite. It's what is also sometimes referred to as emotional eating.

When you're eating for any reason other than physical hunger, that's typically what is labeled "emotional eating." It doesn't mean you're emotional. It means you're feeling something other than hunger or that your appetite has triggered you to eat. What you're feeling other than a physical hunger pain might be sadness. It could be fear or anxiety. It might be boredom or feeling nostalgic or even just being happy.

An easy way to know the difference between an emotion that triggers appetite, or the desire to eat, and true hunger is how specific your cravings are.

Emotional eating is often alleviated only by consuming something you specifically crave, like salty chips, french fries, chocolate, pastry, etc. It can even be healthy, like a big salad at your favorite place for lunch.

Emotional hunger triggers our emotional appetite. It's why you feel like you have to eat something sweet after dinner. You know you're not truly hungry, but you still have this feeling, and we'll often say, "Oh, I'm really craving," or "I'm hungry for something sweet." It's that feeling of dissatisfaction even after you've eaten a meal, and that feeling is an emotion, because all feelings are part of our emotions.

Your CTA:

How often were you truly hungry today, and how often was it appetite? Write it down in your journal.

_____
_____
_____
_____
_____
_____
_____
_____
_____
_____
_____
_____
_____
_____
_____
_____
_____
_____
_____
_____
_____
_____
_____
_____
_____
_____
_____

"What else are you hungry for?"

_____
_____
_____
_____
_____
_____
_____
_____
_____
_____
_____
_____
_____
_____
_____
_____
_____
_____
_____
_____
_____
_____
_____
_____
_____
_____
_____

Day 11

Do you have a dieter's mentality? It's an all-or-nothing mindset with only two options: perfection or failure. This mindset is common for people when they're starting a new journey, especially diets.

For so many of us, this mentality stems from childhood.

Maybe you had critical parents or felt internal pressure to be perfect. If things didn't go perfectly, you quit or felt like you were a failure. Perhaps you never start, because never starting means you can never fail.

Perfection doesn't exist, and nobody wants to fail, so we create alternatives to avoid failure. What do we do? We never start. Those are the people who are obsessed with making sure everything is right and the timing is perfect before they start changing their diet. "I'm going to start exercising after vacation" or "I'm going to clean out the pantry after our company leaves" or "I might as well wait until next month, next Monday, next year," etc. We have many reasons why it's not the right time to make a change.

The second alternative is quitting. Maybe you had a bad day or you ate something you're bummed out about because you know you didn't need it and now you feel bad. Rather than treating it as just a slip, you turn it into a slippery slope and quit dieting. Why? You weren't perfect, and you don't want to consider yourself a failure, so you stop and make excuses, like you quit because you weren't feeling well. You slipped because you didn't have enough information or support from your family.

We make excuses when the truth is we're just afraid to fail. No place is that more true than in your journey to health.

You want to be the best YOU possible. To do that, you've got to drop the dieter's mentality. Get rid of that all-or-nothing thinking. This is about progress. Yes, you're going to have a few bad days. Yes, you're going to have a meal you wish you hadn't eaten. It's no big deal. Correct it with the next meal, not the next day, week, month, or year.

Don't throw in the towel. Don't beat yourself up. Give yourself some grace.

Success happens when we recognize the progress we're making. Each one of those failures, each experiment we do, each time we look at ourselves and say, "You know what? I did my best and I can do better," that's progress, so drop the dieter's mentality. You're making progress every day. You are a success.

Your CTA for today:

Notice throughout the day when you have any thoughts about achieving perfection or quitting. When it happens, say to yourself, "I know what I don't want. What is it that I do?"

_____

_____

_____

_____

_____

_____

_____

_____

_____

_____

_____

_____

_____

_____

_____

_____

_____

_____

_____

_____

_____

_____

_____

_____

_____

"*No more diets*"

Day 12

Slow down and experience your meals.

The twenty-minute meal is important. This is one I'm constantly working on, as a hairstylist, salon owner, personal trainer, health coach, and busy mom, I'm eating on the run all the time, which doesn't help later, when I'm having dinner with my family.

Bottom line, I'm a fast eater.

When I first tried this twenty-minute meal, I was going crazy at how slow it was.

Here's the importance of it though: it is part of being present and aware of your meals. It gives your stomach time to tell your brain you are full, so you don't overeat.

Digestion starts in the mouth. As we chew our food, enzymes are released, telling our stomach to get ready; food is coming.

When we chew our food long enough, the enzymes released in our mouth also tell our stomach we are very satisfied with our meal.

You have a few CTAs for today:

Time one of your meals at your regular speed.

On your next meal, try to get to twenty minutes. If you eat your meal in five minutes, this may be really hard at first. Maybe try adding five-minute increments on your next meals.

Things to focus on:

- Do the 5-5-7 breathing exercise before you eat, if you are even remotely stressed.
- Chew your food a total of fifteen to twenty-five chews before you swallow.
- Put your fork down between bites.
- Put your phone down, so you are not distracted.

My husband makes amazing meals that are both aesthetically lovely and delicious. Every time he sets food in front of me, I start doing a little shimmy dance in my chair, and then after I take a bite, I do the same thing.

It really just happened naturally the first time, but when we are positive, present, and aware when we are eating, we get to experience our food in a whole new way.

Have you ever been on vacation and all the food tasted better? When we are on vacation we are usually more relaxed, taking in all the new surroundings and in the present moment. That's why our meals taste better.

I remember being in Aruba after a long travel day getting there. It was nighttime. I couldn't see the turquoise waters of the Caribbean, but I could smell and hear the waves crashing and taste the saltwater in the air, excited to be somewhere I'd never been. There was a cute outdoor restaurant at the hotel lit up by candles on the table and lights strung overhead. We ordered a charcuterie board and wine. It was one of the best meals of my life. You guys, it was only meat, cheese, crackers, and dried fruits. I experienced that meal with ALL my senses.

I remember another time that food was out of this world when I had a cup of coffee and pastry one afternoon in San Francisco with my mom, twenty-three years ago. We were sitting outside on a gorgeous day, looking out at the bay, overlooking the Golden Gate Bridge. I remember birds flying around and all the people were enjoying their time. Was it really the most amazing chocolate croissant and coffee? Possibly, but maybe not. The EXPERIENCE I had made it that way.

I've had many similar experiences while on vacations or even quick weekend getaways up to the mountains, or wherever. I try to have those experiences with my meals often. Some days stress and a fast-paced society get the best of me.

Your CTA for today is to eat with ALL your senses.

Sight: is your food appealing?

Sound: what are you hearing around you?

Smell: close your eyes and see if you can smell a specific herb or spice.

Taste: digestion starts in the mouth, so chew your food rather than two chomps and then a swallow.

Touch: I'm not telling you to eat your soup with your hands, but if you're eating something that doesn't use utensils, pay attention to the food you touch, even as you are preparing it.

_____

_____

_____

_____

_____

_____

_____

_____

_____

_____

_____

_____

_____

_____

_____

_____

_____

_____

_____

_____

"Your senses are magical"

Day 13

Every symptom, craving, or behavior around food has a positive intention. Therefore, symptoms, cravings, or behaviors are not the problem. They are just the best solution you have come up with so far. They are a messenger that's asking you to seek a new solution.

Cravings are your body's request for balance. What needs to be balanced in your life?

Your body always has positive intentions. It has inherant wisdom beyond any force.

"Nourishment" is about much more than food; what we take in all day is "food."

- Chaos in the morning with your family is "food" you're taking in.
- Traffic frustration is "food."
- Negative talk at work is "food."
- Negative talk in the mirror is "food."

There is a saying that I love so much, "How you do one thing is how you do everything."

At first I didn't understand it, and then all of a sudden it clicked. When my house feels chaotic and cluttered, when I'm in a funk, when my car is a disaster, when I'm fighting with my loved ones or just being negative, my food choices are not great and my workouts suffer.

Nourish your words, your actions, yourself with good, positive intentions at all times.

Love where you're at NOW, not where you want to be.

No matter how much weight you want to lose, stop looking in the mirror with negative thoughts. Stop stepping on the scale with disgust and disappointment.

Buy clothes that fit you well, wear bright and fun colors, style your hair, paint your nails, buy a bright lipstick, and ROCK YOUR BODY NOW.

We tend to get into a "when I lose such and such amount of weight, I'm going to _____."

Basically you're holding off your life until you have a different body.

Look in the mirror.

What do you see?

Are you strong?

Are you beautiful?

Are you ALIVE?

Did you birth babies?

Do you have curves?

What has that body done for you?

Where has it carried you?

Your CTA for today:

Stand naked in front of the mirror and scan your body. No negative talk here.

What do you love?

How can you nourish yourself?

The point of this exercise is all part of being in the present moment, appreciating where you are, meeting yourself where you are NOW, and loving that person looking back at you. It's all important for your overall health.

You can't have all this outside work to be done if you haven't done anything on the inside.

Write down what this all means to you and the first thing you'll do to take action.

"What 'foods' are you taking in all day?"

_____
_____
_____
_____
_____
_____
_____
_____
_____
_____
_____
_____
_____
_____
_____
_____
_____
_____
_____
_____
_____
_____
_____
_____
_____
_____
_____
_____
_____
_____

Day 14

Meal breakdown as a guideline and "kitchen closed after dinner" mantra

Try this for a few days and see if it jives with you:

First thing when you get up, your body is dehydrated, so don't drink that coffee until you've had sixteen ounces of water

Breakfast:
Sixteen ounces of water before anything else.
Your breakfast plate should be high protein, with a fiber-filled (complex) carb and a healthy fat to give you energy and fill you until lunch.
Your plate should be 50 percent protein, 50 percent healthy carbs

Lunch:
Sixteen ounces of water first.
Lunch should be mainly veggies, with protein and a little bit of complex carbs and a little healthy fat. This will give you the energy you need to finish out the day.
Your plate should be 50 percent vegetables, 25 percent protein and 25 percent complex carbs.

Snack: (optional)
Sixteen ounces of water first
Vegetables and a little protein and/or healthy fat

Dinner:
Sixteen ounces of water first

By this point, you no longer need the complex carbs for energy, unless you are carb loading for a race or really intense workout the next morning. Your dinner plate should be 75 percent vegetables and 25 percent protein.

Here are some things you can easily incorporate into your lifestyle. The hardest change is if you're used to high-carb dinners.

You can replace these veggies for your carbs:

- 👈 Romaine lettuce boats for tortilla/taco shells or buns
- 👈 Cauliflower "rice" for rice
- 👈 Sweet potato or turnip for white potato
- 👈 Zoodles (zucchini noodles) or cabbage for pasta

Kitchen closed after dinner. Period. No if's, ands, or but's about it. There are a few reasons why we eat after dinner:

1. Habit
2. Boredom
3. Didn't eat enough during the day and you are famished

After-dinner snacking calories can add up quickly. Your spouse, kids, or loved ones are snacking, and you lose willpower. All of a sudden your well-planned, healthy day just turned into 200 to 500 calories over what you wanted it to be.

After-dinner snacking was one of my biggest downfalls years ago. I stopped the after-dinner snacking, and it made a positive impact on my nutrition. I am not perfect with my meals, but one thing I do is follow the mantra "kitchen closed after dinner."

Making sure you get enough filling foods throughout the day will really help with after-dinner cravings.

If it's a habit and you're really not hungry, try having a cup of tea or glass of seltzer water with some berries or citrus. Using your favorite mug or wine glass, make it an evening ritual. You can also try distracting your after-dinner snacking habit with a walk, writing in your journal, meditation, a bath, painting your nails, knitting, reading, etc.

Your CTA: would you like to try this?

"Kitchen closed after dinner"

Day 15

Think of your body as a savings account.

If you continue to withdraw nutrients by eating refined sugar and not replacing it with nutrient-dense foods, your body becomes depleted, which can lead to all sorts of health issues.

Let's take carbs for an example.

Simple carbs (white flour, sugar, white rice, etc.) digest quickly

vs.

Complex carbs (whole grains, beans, fruit, etc.) digest slowly

When complex carbs are processed or refined, they deplete our body's reserve of vitamins and minerals. For example, if you take whole wheat and turn it into a bagel, the wheat gets stripped of fiber and nutrients, to be turned into flour. The bagel becomes a simple carb, which spikes blood sugar. Your brain and your body turn it into an "emergency situation" that prompts the pancreas to produce insulin. All of a sudden it's too much, and then you crash.

That, my friends, is the blood sugar roller-coaster.

It causes enormous stress, both biological and chemical, on the body.

Physical effects of sugar:

- A weakened immune system, which destroys germ-killing ability of white blood cells for up to five hours after digestion
- Type two diabetes: insulin receptors no longer respond to insulin produced in the pancreas, and cells are less able to get energy from food we eat
- Hypoglycemia: fatigue, lack of concentration, mood swings, shaking, sweating

- Depression: messes with serotonin levels
- Increased cancer risk: pancreas, skin, womb, urinary tract, and breast cancer under the age of forty-nine
- Weight gain: excess sugar stores as fat. When your body is producing insulin it can't produce glucagon. Its function is to take fat out of storage to be burned.

Counting chemicals trumps counting calories.
Eat more rather than less:
More high-quality foods
More seasonal and organic foods
More foods that grow
More shopping the perimeter of the grocery store

Look at labels and choose foods with few ingredients and ingredients you can actually pronounce.

If you want something such as potato chips, choose kettle chips made with very few ingredients over canned chips made with more than twenty-five ingredients, including some you can't even pronounce.

Be a label-reading pro.

When you feed your body REAL food, your body knows what to do with it.

It knows how to process that food.

When you feed your body chemicals, it goes into a bit of shock because it doesn't recognize it.

Your CTA for today:

Go to your pantry and fridge, look at labels, and see if there's anything that can be replaced with something better.

What did you find?

Your sugar CTA: Any time you reach for sugar, stop and look at it with those things in mind. Do you still eat it? Honestly, sometimes we do, but knowledge is power. A little bit once in a while is fine. Daily intake and lots of sweet treats too often derail the results you are looking for.

_____

_____

_____

_____

_____

_____

_____

_____

_____

_____

_____

_____

_____

_____

_____

_____

_____

_____

"Counting chemicals trumps counting calories"

Day 16

Inflammation is a huge part of the issue with the foods we are eating or not eating. Take a look at these lists and start shifting your foods to the more anti-inflammatory choices. Also note if you have a sensitivity to anything that might not agree with you. Keep track of all the foods you are eating.

Increase your diet of these anti-inflammatory foods:
Non-starchy vegetables
Extra virgin olive oil
Avocado oil
Raw nuts and seeds
Lemons and limes
Grass-fed, grass-finished beef
MCT oil
Bone broth
Whole eggs
Wild caught salmon
Berries
Avocados
Ghee
Unrefined coconut oil

Experiment on yourself, as these foods may be inflammatory for SOME people, while tolerated by others
Inflammatory "maybe" foods:
Eggs
Kombucha
Caffeine
Chocolate

Beans
Vinegars
Dairy
Grains
Stevia
Citrus fruit
Coffee
Some nuts
Carbonated beverages
Guar or xanthan gums
Organic fermented soy
Nightshade vegetables (tomatoes, white potatoes, peppers, eggplant, tomatillos, okra, gogi berries)

These are foods that should be avoided for a lot of people because of their inflammatory effects.

Inflammatory foods:
Gluten
Alcohol
Grains
Dairy
Soy
Peanuts
Soda
Fast food
Fried foods
Artificial colors or dyes
Sugar
High fructose corn syrup
Artificial sweeteners
Vegetable oils
Smoked, canned, or processed meats

Refined carbohydrates
Jams, jellies, syrups
Hydrogenated oils
"Fruit" beverages, not 100 percent juice
Conventionally raised animal foods

Your CTA for today:

Make a list of foods you eat that could possibly be causing inflammation in your body. Your gut health is the most important thing to your overall health. You are your body's best advocate.

Do you notice any gut issues when you eat certain foods? You may need to eliminate them for a healthier body and lifestyle.

_____
_____
_____
_____
_____
_____
_____
_____
_____
_____
_____
_____
_____
_____
_____
_____
_____
_____
_____
_____
_____
_____

"You are your body's best advocate"

Day 17

We've all "self-medicated" with food before. I don't know one single person who hasn't.

We've all been at a point in our lives (maybe even now) when we were searching for something to be fulfilled and trying to fill that void, emptiness, or anxiousness with food. Does it satisfy that feeling of wanting something? What happens?

It might work for some temporarily because it numbs us, but usually it leaves us still wanting. Often it's some part of us that wants to be more expressed but feels suppressed.

It's a sign that something wants our attention.

Perhaps we're working too much and creativity has been put on hold.

Maybe we've been home-bodying too much and we want more social time with our friends, but instead of recognizing the message in this "hunger," we only recognize the feelings of dissatisfaction or anxiety and quickly turn to food to medicate ourselves. This is an obsession. Can you relate?

Here's the thing: there is a gift in this obsession. Any obsession we have is a powerful HEALING opportunity. It is the body trying to communicate a need or desire, usually some place in our lives where we are under expressed.

The body pretty much tells us at all times exactly what we need.

This is our innate wisdom.

We have just forgotten how to listen for what we really want in that moment. Any time we feel ANXIOUS, BORED, DEPRESSED, or FRUSTRATED, or any time we feel bad about ourselves, judge our bodies, or even feel pain and we reach for food to self-medicate, it's time to step back and listen.

Underneath that hunger is usually some area of our life where we'd like to be more expressed or where we need to devote more time and energy.

Your CTA for today:

Journal and get in tune with your body and what you truly want. Does this make sense? What is resonating with you so far? Looking back, can you think of a specific time where this may have been you?

_____

_____

_____

_____

_____

_____

_____

_____

_____

_____

_____

_____

_____

_____

_____

_____

_____

_____

_____

_____

_____

_____

_____

_____

_____

"Food is not the answer to fill a void in your life"

_____

_____

_____

_____

_____

_____

_____

_____

_____

_____

_____

_____

_____

_____

_____

_____

_____

_____

_____

_____

_____

_____

_____

_____

_____

_____

_____

_____

Day 18

Mental fitness and inner fitness

I want to focus on mental fitness. Mental fitness means keeping your brain and emotional health in tip-top shape. Keeping your mind mentally fit is as easy as taking time out of your busy day to do the following:

- Meditate/be mindful
- Read
- Daydream

Some other ways to keep yourself mentally fit include the following:

- Stop multitasking - I admit I am a multitasker. We often think that multitasking enables us to get more things done at once, but it actually creates more problems than it solves. Focusing on one task at a time improves our concentration and helps us be more productive.
- Positivity - Positivity breeds positive change. Daily positive affirmations are a great way to get your day started in a positive manner each day. Affirmation, or talking to yourself in a positive way, involves strengthening neural pathways to bring your self-confidence, well-being, and satisfaction to a higher level. It raises your vibration and helps manifest more positivity.

To start, make a list of your good qualities and the things you want to work on. Next write positive statements regarding each quality you either have already or are striving for. Here are some of mine:

-- I am patient. I don't react to any situation before I take a moment to breathe and process.
-- I am productive. I am productive and focused in everything I do.
-- I am kind. I treat others with the kindness with which I would like to be treated.

☛ Sleep - Sleep should actually be in the #1 spot. If we aren't getting adequate sleep, we aren't ever going to be mentally fit. Are you getting good sleep each night? If you are chronically getting less than six to seven hours of sleep each night, the rest of your fitness will suffer. For a long time I was getting only about six hours on most nights, and I could tell my body needed more. I've made a conscious choice to get to bed earlier each night to allow for seven hours minimum.

-- Good sleep habits:

  ▪ Bed is for sleeping and sex. Your brain needs to know what it's supposed to do when your head hits that pillow. That means no reading or TV in bed. If you must read to fall asleep, that's fine, but do it in a cozy chair in your room, close to your bed.

  ▪ Turn off electronics at least one hour before bed. The blue light of our phones, computers, and TVs activates our brains and makes falling asleep more difficult and results in a restless night of sleep.

  ▪ Stop eating/drinking at least two hours before bed. The act of digestion is enough to keep us awake, and the blood sugar ups and downs create restlessness, especially when it comes to alcohol close to bedtime.

Your CTA today:

Take action on any/all of those things above. Imperfect action is better
than no action at all.

_____
_____
_____
_____
_____
_____
_____
_____
_____
_____
_____
_____
_____
_____
_____
_____
_____
_____
_____
_____
_____
_____
_____
_____
_____
_____

"Imperfect action is still action"

_____
_____
_____
_____
_____
_____
_____
_____
_____
_____
_____
_____
_____
_____
_____
_____
_____
_____
_____
_____
_____
_____
_____
_____
_____
_____

Day 19

We are not garbage disposals.

How many times do you take a bite of the rest of your kids' french toast as you are walking it to the trash? Taste the dough when you are making cookies? Finish the rest of the mac and cheese in the pot because there's not enough to save for later?

"You don't want it to go to waste..."
"Finish your dinner..."
"There are people starving in _____"

Most of us grew up with our parents saying this stuff to us. Our brains are wired after all those years to WANT, HAVE, and NEED to eat the rest of whatever it is. Those habits took root, and now we are paying attention to it. Release those roots and do something different.

If you're full, push your plate away.

If you have goals, and eating the rest of your kids' food on their plate doesn't align with them, don't eat it. Throw it away, store it for later, for them, but don't eat it!

These little shifts will make HUGE changes in the long run. Be aware of your choices first and then choose to DO SOMETHING DIFFERENT.

Have you ever felt like you've overeaten, over-treated, or are stumbling or struggling in one way or another?
Things to remember:
You are always learning.
As long as you are present, you are on track.

You can always lose weight as fast as you can gain weight.

You never, ever need to wait till Monday, the first of the month, or a new year to get it together.

It's never too late to drink more water, write down your meals and feelings, learn and reflect, and make a better plan for your next meal.

When you slip, think about why it happened and how you would have done it differently. Face it head on, not head in the sand. Look at a slip with curiosity and WITHOUT judgment.

Even if it felt like a rare event, history repeats itself, and you want to be better prepared mentally and physically for success in the future.

Your CTA for today:

Pay attention to every little bite, taste, and nibble you WANT to take, but choose NOT to. If you happen to have a slip, write down your experience.

_____

_____

_____

_____

_____

_____

_____

_____

_____

_____

_____

_____

_____

_____

_____

_____

_____

_____

_____

_____

_____

_____

_____

_____

_____

_____

"Curiosity over judgment"

_____
_____
_____
_____
_____
_____
_____
_____
_____
_____
_____
_____
_____
_____
_____
_____
_____
_____
_____
_____
_____
_____
_____
_____
_____
_____
_____
_____

Day 20

To weigh or not to weigh

This is a biggie. Are you a scale junkie? Is using a scale helpful to keep you motivated? Does it derail you and depress you?

Figure out what your relationship is going to be with the scale.

Take measurements to see your progress; they are incredibly important.

How do you FEEL about the scale?

There are several options for using the scale as a tool. That is all it is—a tool. It does not tell you your worth or who you are as a person.

Some people find it most beneficial to weigh every day. If this idea resonates with you, the best thing to do is weigh yourself first thing in the morning after you go to the restroom. Either go nude or wear the same thing every time. This method works for people who like to know every day where they are. It may help keep you on track with your choices throughout the day.

Others may find that a once-a-week weigh-in helps them. This method may be beneficial for you if you get a little obsessed with the number on the scale. A once-a-week weigh-in helps to show more pounds lost in total and not daily fluctuations.

Others may have to not weigh at all, burn their scale, or bury it six feet under. If you get really down, depressed, or angry with the numbers, stop the madness and get rid of the scale altogether. Go with how you feel in your clothes and take measurements once a month.

Side note: If you are doing an intense weight training program, please do not get discouraged with the scale.

I've heard it many times, and it actually makes me a little crazy when people say "muscle weighs more than fat." A pound of muscle and a pound of fat both weigh a pound. Muscle is more dense than fat; therefore, a pound of muscle will take up much less room in your body than a pound of fat. You may not lose all that much weight, but you'll be surprised with inches lost.

Your CTA today:

Which resonates with you the most regarding the scale and measurements? Do that.

_____

_____

_____

_____

_____

_____

_____

_____

_____

_____

_____

_____

_____

_____

_____

_____

_____

_____

_____

_____

_____

_____

_____

_____

_____

_____

"*The scale shows only your gravitational pull to the ground*"

_____
_____
_____
_____
_____
_____
_____
_____
_____
_____
_____
_____
_____
_____
_____
_____
_____
_____
_____
_____
_____
_____
_____
_____
_____
_____
_____

Day 21

Measuring progress. Take a look back at the last twenty-one days.

Progress can be physical:

Weight loss
Inches lost
More energy
Better sleep
Dropping a dress size
Clothes fitting better
Exercising with greater ease
Working out longer
Working out with more intensity
Fewer aches and pains

Progress can be psychological:

More confident in your skin
Less anxious in uncomfortable situations
Limiting yourself to one dessert or one glass of wine
Conquering an emotional trigger
Eating a mindful meal
Feeling empowered to make healthy choices
Feeling darned good in life

Progress can be social:

Being more social

Compliments from others
Choosing a healthier entree at a restaurant
Resisting temptations at the grocery store
Turning down treats at work
Saying no to a food pusher
Getting your family/friends on the health train

Progress can be whatever the heck YOU want it to be:

Meal prepping for the week
Cooking a new recipe
Bringing your lunch to work
Trying a new healthy food
Developing a distaste for unhealthy food
Cooking at home instead of eating or ordering out
Craving healthy foods
Taking the stairs more often
Changing your commute
Staying in your calorie range consistently
Easily getting all your steps in for the day

Just remember: if weight loss is your goal and you're making progress on some of these items, eventually you WILL lose weight. You just have to keep going and be consistent.

Your CTA for today:

Write out all of your progress.

_____

_____

_____

_____

_____

_____

_____

_____

_____

_____

_____

_____

_____

_____

_____

_____

_____

_____

_____

_____

_____

_____

_____

_____

_____

_____

_____

_____

_____

_____

_____

"Forward progression will always move you forward"

_____
_____
_____
_____
_____
_____
_____
_____
_____
_____
_____
_____
_____
_____
_____
_____
_____
_____
_____
_____
_____
_____
_____
_____
_____
_____
_____

Day 22

Why is the late afternoon/evening harder when it comes to making healthy choices?

When it comes to 3:00 in the afternoon or when it gets to Friday, sometimes we end up with zero willpower and reach for something unhealthy. We may justify it as a "reward" for a day/week well done. Sometimes it feels like we truly can't help it; we have to have it.

That is our tired brain, which has made many decisions throughout the day/week. It's on 24/7. There's a part of our brain that, after feeding ourselves sugar/flour at that time of day, thinks it needs it. Sugar/flour spikes your blood sugar, which triggers the "feel good" hormone. You get an endorphin rush and the brain is satisfied and happy, but not for long. We then spiral into that blood sugar rollercoaster, wanting more sugar. Ugh! How do we get out of this?

You CAN overpower that small area of your brain by building the habit to keep saying no. The more you say no, the easier it becomes. YOU are in control of everything you put in your mouth. All you have to do is think, slow down, and keep steering in the right direction. You will slip; you will fail; you will cave in to cravings. Keep pulling yourself up, not beating yourself up.

Focus on progress, not perfection.

Your CTA for today:

What is your biggest struggle with your nutrition? Where are you seeing a "bad" habit, and where have you improved?

_____

_____

_____

_____

_____

_____

_____

_____

_____

_____

_____

_____

_____

_____

_____

_____

_____

_____

_____

_____

_____

_____

_____

_____

_____

_____

"You are exactly where you need to be right now"

Day 23

Do you ever feel like you can't stop eating, like you're never satisfied? This scenario happened to me once when I was feeling really stressed with my son. I went to the pantry, saw gummy bears (I don't even like gummy bears), opened the bag, and grabbed a handful. I poured myself a glass of wine and grabbed a few chunks of cheese.

Put yourself in the same situation. There's no judgment here. You go to the fridge or pantry for a snack. I want you simply to get curious. What are you feeling or craving?

Try filling in the statement "I feel _____because/when _____. I want _____."

My blanks that night would have been "I feel empty because I'm stressed and I feel like a horrible mom. I want something to make me happy."

I was even saying to myself, "This will not make me feel better; this will not help my stress; this will not fill the void. My brain got the better of me and I did it anyway.

What we want to do today is find a way to get what you want/need without self-destruction. We are going for non-edible nourishing ways to meet your emotional needs or cravings.

Personal nourishment:

Here are some things you can do for personal nourishment, rather than reaching for chips, alcohol, and/or chocolate. See if doing one of these would help.

Massage

Yoga
Dance
Music
Shower/bath with lit candles
Green drink
Facial
Manicure or pedicure
Sensual pleasure
Flowers
House cleaner
Warm blanket out of the dryer
Meditate
Write in gratitude journal
Deep conversation
Organizing something
Writing a letter to a loved one
Anything else you can think of

Your CTA today:

Make a nourishment list. What will be your go-to for a non-self-destructive path?

_____

_____

_____

_____

_____

_____

_____

_____

_____

_____

_____

_____

_____

_____

_____

_____

_____

_____

_____

_____

_____

_____

_____

_____

"Self-care is not selfish"

Day 24

New goals and reflection. What positive things have you accomplished in the last twenty-four days?

It's time to write some new goals. Those goals need to be

S. Specific
M. Measurable
A. Attainable
R. Relevant
T. Time bound

Writing your goals on a piece of paper is the number-one way to help you reach them.

First and foremost we need to PRAISE our accomplishments, and then we need to sit quietly and figure out what we want next.

Is there an area that we could have done better?

One of the best quotes from the creator of Whole 30 program is this:

This is not hard. Don't you dare tell us this is hard. Fighting cancer is hard. Birthing a baby is hard. Losing a parent is hard. Drinking your coffee black. Is. Not. Hard. You've done harder things than this, and you have no excuse not to complete the program as written. It's only thirty days, and it's for the most important health cause on earth—the only physical body you will own.

Your Big Motivating factor:
What's your big Motivating Factor?
What is the desired outcome you want to see?

We really have to figure out the driving force of WHY we want that outcome, the WHY that makes you cry. What is having that thing going to do for you? What are you fighting for and WHY?

Your CTA for today:

Write some short-term and long-term goals. What do you desire in 10 years, 5 years, 1 year, 1 month, and tomorrow? Start with your 10 year plan and work backwards.

_____

_____

_____

_____

_____

_____

_____

_____

_____

_____

_____

_____

_____

_____

_____

_____

_____

_____

_____

_____

_____

_____

_____

_____

_____

"Your why that makes you cry"

Day 25

Honor hunger and fullness.

If you want to build healthy habits around food, WHAT you eat is only part of the big picture. We also have to look at:

HOW we eat (fast, slow, distracted, stressed, etc.)

WHO you are being when you eat

Do you eat when you're not actually hungry?

Do you eat too little or too much?

How do you "honor hunger?"

Tune into your internal signal that the body needs nourishment.

Recognize hunger—learn the signs.

Create an intuitive inner scale from one to ten. One is just noticing hunger; ten is starving.

Start to plan food when you are at a two.

How do you "honor fullness?"

Create a fullness scale from one to ten. Ten is stuffed; one is still starving. It takes twenty minutes for your stomach to tell your brain that you are full. We discussed the twenty-minute meal on day 12.

Aim for a seven on the fullness scale—nourished and energized; satiated but not stuffed.

Here are 6 ways you can practice honoring your inner intuitive hunger and fullness scale:

1. Start planning what and when to eat when you are at a level two on the hunger/fullness scale.
2. Eat high energy foods that your body wants.

3. Eat for energy (aim for a level seven on your inner intuitive scale versus a level ten, where you're so full you have to unzip your pants)

4. Make a physical gesture that your meal is complete by pushing your plate away, putting your napkin over it, crossing your silverware, or even putting some ice cubes on it.

5. Declare out loud to yourself or whomever you're with that you are full. This acknowledgment will dissuade you from continuing to eat, because you've already announced that the meal was complete for you.

6. If you're out, get a box for leftovers as soon as your plate comes to the table and put half your meal in the box immediately. Restaurants serve huge portions, so getting rid of half and saving it for another meal will automatically save you hundreds of extra calories.

Your CTA for today:

Write this down in your journal and repeat it out loud daily:

"I set up the CONDITIONS for success in my life so that FOLLOW-THROUGH happens."

_____

_____

_____

_____

_____

_____

_____

_____

_____

_____

_____

_____

_____

_____

_____

_____

_____

_____

_____

_____

_____

_____

_____

_____

_____

_____

_____

"I honor my hunger and fullness with presence and love"

_____
_____
_____
_____
_____
_____
_____
_____
_____
_____
_____
_____
_____
_____
_____
_____
_____
_____
_____
_____
_____
_____
_____
_____
_____
_____
_____

Day 26

Habits: Automatic and Keystone

An automatic habit is something you do automatically. It's a regular tendency or practice, with almost no thought required.

You make habits by repeating a behavior over and over and over to solidify it in your brain.

There are also keystone habits. Keystone habits are small changes that unintentionally carry over into other aspects of your life. They create a domino effect that changes all areas of your life.

A keystone habit is a habit you do that helps other habits fall into place.

A great example of a keystone habit is meal prepping.

When you meal prep, you've got your meals and snacks set for the week.

At lunch, while your coworkers are eating fast food, you've got your low-caloric density meal to keep you satisfied.

When you need that afternoon pick-me-up, you have the carrots, crackers, and hummus you brought from home so you can steer clear of the chips and sweets in the breakroom.

How'd you make those healthy choices?

Simple: meal prepping, a great keystone habit that leads to other great habits.

Writing and tracking your meals in your journal is a great keystone habit that helps lead you to success with your nutritional choices.

Your CTA:

What automatic daily habits do you already have in place, and what keystone habits do you practice?

_____

_____

_____

_____

_____

_____

_____

_____

_____

_____

_____

_____

_____

_____

_____

_____

_____

_____

_____

_____

_____

_____

_____

_____

_____

_____

" You are what your habits are"

_____
_____
_____
_____
_____
_____
_____
_____
_____
_____
_____
_____
_____
_____
_____
_____
_____
_____
_____
_____
_____
_____
_____
_____
_____
_____
_____
_____
_____

Day 27

Meal planning 101

Meal planning avoids having to use willpower. We love having a ton of choices, yet those choices can stress us out and lead us to decision fatigue. All the food decisions you make throughout the day can slowly chip away at your willpower, but planning your meals in advance can keep you from having to rely on willpower in the first place. Planning your meals may take a little extra effort one day a week, but it means you'll know exactly what to reach for the next time you're hungry. You can save all that leftover willpower for when you really need it.

Great reasons to meal plan and prep:

1. You'll make better food choices.

The idea of having infinite options sounds great in theory, but when you're exhausted and hungry and you don't have a game plan, you'll probably just end up making the same old fallback meal or ordering the usual takeout. "Throwing something together" will usually lead to unbalanced meals. After all, it's hard to make healthy choices when you're hungry. Perhaps you'll even make dinner while drinking wine and snacking on cheese and crackers that will probably fill you up before your meal, yet you'll eat the whole meal anyway.

Meal planning and prepping helps you get all those decisions out of the way at once while you're still feeling relaxed, recharged, and motivated.

2. You'll cut back on mindless snacking.

You're hungry for a snack, so you grab a handful of almonds...and then another...and then another. Before you know it, you're halfway through the tin, and your "healthy" snack has tacked on a few hundred extra calories. When you're hungry, stressed, or tired, it's easy to eat mindlessly and give into cravings.

3. You'll make room in your schedule for other things.

Yes, there's a time commitment. Whatever day you decide to meal prep for the week, you'll invest a few hours planning your schedule, shopping for healthy ingredients, and batch-prepping your meals, but after that, you won't waste time before every single meal rummaging through the kitchen, trying to figure out what to cook.

Your CTA today:

If you are already prepping your meals, please continue. If it is new for you, get going. What day will you grocery shop and meal prep?

_____
_____
_____
_____
_____
_____
_____
_____
_____
_____
_____
_____
_____
_____
_____
_____
_____
_____
_____
_____
_____
_____
_____
_____
_____

"A failure to plan is a plan to fail"

_____

_____

_____

_____

_____

_____

_____

_____

_____

_____

_____

_____

_____

_____

_____

_____

_____

_____

_____

_____

_____

_____

_____

_____

Day 28

Grit, Willpower and Core Beliefs

Don't focus on yesterday's mistakes; focus on today's goals.

When you're trying to lose weight, it's easy to obsess over the occasional slip-up—a high-calorie snack here, a skipped workout there—and lose sight of your long-term goals. But the ability to rally after a setback is more important than the ability to make virtuous decisions all the time.

Grit is staying focused on a long-term goal, come hell or high water. You are firm and fearless. You have to dig deep for grit and remember your WHY.

Willpower is the ability to control yourself. It is your strong determination that allows you to do something difficult.

The next time you're tempted to curse your lack of willpower, remember that self-control is a skill, and like any skill, you'll screw up a few times while you're learning it. What's important is that you keep going.

Determine your weak areas or obstacles and make a plan to overcome them. Put your plan into practice, evaluate it, and adjust it if necessary. Expect to stray from the plan occasionally and know that you can keep moving forward. Eating fast food doesn't make you bad at following a healthy nutrition lifestyle any more than having a fender bender makes you a bad driver.

We need to get rid of the shaming, guilt, and judgment.

Core beliefs are basic beliefs about ourselves, others, and the world we live in. They are things we hold to be rooted truths to the core of our being. Core beliefs can be both positive and negative. The more we uphold and focus on our positive and healthy core beliefs, the more we can overshadow and release the negative ones.

Your CTA for today:

No matter what is happening today, replace any negative thought with something loving. What did you do yesterday that you will bless and release with love? What is ONE thing you will focus on TODAY that will get you closer to your goal?

_____

_____

_____

_____

_____

_____

_____

_____

_____

_____

_____

_____

_____

_____

_____

_____

_____

_____

_____

_____

_____

_____

_____

_____

"I don't have time in my life for guilt and judgment"

_____

_____

_____

_____

_____

_____

_____

_____

_____

_____

_____

_____

_____

_____

_____

_____

_____

_____

_____

_____

_____

_____

_____

_____

_____

_____

_____

Day 29

The Importance of Self Confidence

To achieve even the smallest of goals and get through life's daily duties and responsibilities, you have to have some self-confidence. A self-confident attitude allows you to wade through the push and pull of different voices and opinions telling you, "yes, no, maybe, do this, do that," etc. Relying on other people to guide you and following their opinions robs you of your individuality, makes you unsure of yourself, and can lead to depression.

DEFINITION

Self-confidence is an attitude you hold about yourself that allows you to move forward and achieve your goals. It is having a positive attitude, with realistic views. Self-confidence is having a general sense of control of your life, knowing that you can do what you desire. Self-confidence means that even if things don't go your way, you still believe that eventually, somehow, some way, they will.

DEVELOPING SELF CONFIDENCE

When you were young your parents may have instilled self-confidence in you by encouraging self-reliance and giving you love, even when you made mistakes. If you did not have your parents' help, you can develop self-confidence yourself by mastering the ability to feel certain you really can achieve something.

VISUALIZE

Sitting quietly with your eyes closed and mentally visualizing yourself in great detail as a confident person is a great way to start being confident. When you repeatedly visualize yourself being and acting confident and achieving what you wish by confidently going after it, you will act confidently because your mind sees confidence as familiar ground.

OVERCOMING NEGATIVE THOUGHTS

There are several strategies to overcoming negative thoughts that keep you trapped in lack of confidence. First, emphasize strengths by giving yourself credit. Second, take risks by looking at new experiences as a chance to learn, not win or lose. Third, use self-talk by stopping in the middle of a negative thought and reframing it with a positive thought or words. Fourth, self-evaluation allows you to gain a stronger sense of self and stop giving away your personal power to others.

MOVE FORWARD WITH CONFIDENCE

Becoming self-confident does not mean you are unrealistic about yourself and your situation. You understand that you are not Superman/woman, but being confident means still moving forward toward achieving your goal and fulfilling your desires, even when things don't seem to be going your way. Using positive self-talk such as "I can do this, I am the best, I've got this, and I have all that I desire," can help you get through times of doubt and help you maintain a feeling of self-confidence.

Your CTA for today:

In what areas do you have self-confidence and what areas need some work?

_____

_____

_____

_____

_____

_____

_____

_____

_____

_____

_____

_____

_____

_____

_____

_____

_____

_____

_____

_____

_____

_____

_____

_____

_____

_____

_____

_____

_____

"I believe in my greatness and personal power"

_____
_____
_____
_____
_____
_____
_____
_____
_____
_____
_____
_____
_____
_____
_____
_____
_____
_____
_____
_____
_____
_____
_____
_____
_____
_____
_____
_____
_____

Day 30

Recap and six lifetime habits to incorporate to become the most vibrant and positive YOU.

I want you to make the impact that's always been there. Like a caterpillar that turns into a butterfly, you are vibrant, strong, and capable of all that you desire.

Lifetime habit # 1

Drink plenty of water. Did you know that water makes up two-thirds of our bodies?

What happens when we are dehydrated? When our cells are under hydrated the body's response is to SLOW down. Our physical performance suffers. We experience headaches and symptoms of fatigue—basically the midday fatigue many of us feel daily.

How do we answer these symptoms?

Oftentimes we turn to caffeine or food.

It's so common that we begin to crave "quick fixes" for our lack of energy when we are under hydrated. What happens next? Those quick fixes use up more of our small supply of body water to be processed, and we dig a deeper hole for ourselves.

Your daily water goal should be half your body weight in ounces, minimum.

Benefits of water:

- GETS RID OF FAT. The process of burning calories requires a good supply of water; dehydration slows down the fat-burning process.

- ☛ GETS RID OF TOXINS. Burning calories creates toxins (think of the exhaust coming out of your car), and water plays a vital role in flushing them out of your body.
- ☛ GIVES ENERGY FOR YOUR WORKOUT. Dehydration causes a reduction in blood volume; which causes a reduction in the supply of oxygen to your muscles. What does that equal? Fatigue, poor performance, and wimpy workouts.

Those facts just break the surface of why water is so vital. Personally, I can tell the difference in my skin when I've had enough water or when I have not.

Lifetime habit #2

Balancing blood sugar is the number-one action to help you resolve digestive issues, heal adrenal fatigue, lose weight, curb cravings, balance hormones, overcome binge and emotional eating, gain energy, stop chronic dieting, fall in love with your body and be comfortable in your own skin, stress less, greatly improve quality of life, look and feel younger, have better sex, and experience deep happiness and satisfaction.

Unfortunately sugar dominates our food supply: crackers, bread, cakes, soda, ketchup, pasta sauce, juice, salad dressings, gum, and even toothpaste can contain sugar.

During sugar production the beet or cane plant is stripped of all fiber and nutrients and turned into the white powder we know. Because sugar has been stripped of any nutrients, your body has to pull on its own reserves of vitamins and minerals to break sugar down.

If you continue to withdraw nutrients from your body by eating refined sugar and not replacing it with nutrient-dense foods, your body becomes depleted. That depletion can lead to all sorts of health risks: weakened immune system, cardiovascular disease, type-two diabetes, hyperglycemia, depression, increased cancer risk, and weight gain.

Example of a good complex carb turned into a simple carb: turning whole wheat into a bagel. The wheat has been stripped of fiber and nutrients and turned into flour. The bagel then turns into a simple carbs that spike blood sugar. Your brain and body turn it into an "emergency situation." Your body alerts the pancreas to increase insulin, and, then there is too much insulin so you get a sugar crash.

That's called the blood-sugar roller-coaster.

It causes enormous stress (biological and chemical) on the body, initiating the stress response on a regular basis, systematically destroying good health.

Counting chemicals trumps counting calories.

Lifetime habit #3

Evaluating the best protein source for your body.

Too little protein can cause crazy sugar cravings; fatigue or feeling weak; hair loss; changing hair color texture; and feeling spacey, jittery, ungrounded, and unfocused.

Too much protein can cause constipation, less-efficient kidney function, bad breath/body odor, weight gain, feeling stiff or tense, and sweets cravings. Also your body can become too acidic and leach calcium from bones to alkalize.

Acidic/alkaline balance: as long as you are eating unprocessed, healthy whole foods and lots of produce, your body will be more alkaline.

I try to eat a little protein with every meal.

Lifetime habit #4 Managing Stress

There is REAL stress and IMAGINED stress. The brain cannot differentiate between the two.

REAL stress: you're going for a hike in the woods and you see a bear. Your heart rate speeds up, blood pressure increases, respiration quickens, and adrenaline, non-adrenaline, and cortisol are released. Blood flow is routed away from digestion because you're not going to want to eat anything while running away from the bear. Blood flow is rerouted to arms and legs because you're going to want to run and get away from the situation as fast as you can. Your digestive system shuts down, and you are in fight-or-flight mode.

IMAGINED stress: stuck in traffic, late for work, trying to get out the door in the morning, trying to meet a deadline, etc. The exact same thing happens in your body as the bear story. Heart rate, blood pressure, and respiration rises. Adrenaline, non-adrenaline, and cortisol are released. Blood flow is routed away from digestion up to arms and legs. Digestive system shuts down.

Do you think your body will accept food and nourish your body in any stressful situation? Probably not.

Solutions: meditating, deep breathing, positive thoughts, looking at your plate of food as nourishment and being thankful for it, and calming your body in stressful situations, especially before you eat.

Lifetime habit #5 Sleep

Having a nighttime routine that gets you to bed early and stress free is key.

Reading, meditating, and/or deep breathing will put you in a calm place to get a good night's sleep. Before your head hits the pillow, turn off your electronic devices at least an hour prior and consume no food or drink two hours prior.

Aim for a seven- to eight-hour goal of sleep each night.

Lifetime habit #6 Movement

Figure out what form of movement and exercise is pleasurable for you.

Do you like yoga, dance, tai chi, pole dancing, boot camp, weight training, running, walking, hiking, riding your bike, Zumba, Pilates?

What sort of movement makes you feel strong, alive, and joyful?

How many times a week do you do it?

What is your motivation for going?

Write down things that are pleasurable for you when it comes to moving your body. Write down what movement you do weekly. Write down what you want to do. Write down what you would do if you "had more time" to do it. Figure out a movement plan and then get moving.

CPSIA information can be obtained
at www.ICGtesting.com
Printed in the USA
FSHW020311200921
84854FS